You Just Have To Lose Weight To Achieve Your Ideal Body:

A 30-day Guide To Total Health And Weight Loss

Elizabeth D. Greene

Want to live a better lifestyle and reduce weight? Check out my weight loss book right away! My book is the ideal resource for anyone trying to improve their health and well-being because it is jam-packed with useful advice, tactics, and healthy lifestyle suggestions for long-term weight loss, as well as motivational anecdotes, professional advice, and expert counsel. My weight loss book offers everything you need to achieve your objectives and sustain a healthy lifestyle for years to come, whether you're trying to lose a few pounds, alter your eating habits, or boost your physical activity. Why then wait? Discover the transformational impact of my weight loss book today as you begin your weight reduction journey!

WISHING YOU ALL THE BEST IN YOUR
WEIGHT LOSS JOURNEY AND BUILDING
A HEALTHY LIVING

INTRODUCTION

In today's world, people are becoming more interested in being in shape, feeling younger, and reducing weight. It may be difficult to know where to begin or what to trust in the health and wellness sector because there are so many divergent trends and viewpoints. "The Truth about Reducing Weight, Being Healthy and Feeling Younger" is a book that addresses these issues. This thorough manual explains how to attain and maintain a healthy weight, excellent health, and a feeling of vitality. It offers evidence-based knowledge and helpful guidance. This book may be an invaluable tool on your path to greater health and well-being, whether your goals are to reduce weight, enhance your general health, or simply feel better about yourself.

Table of content

Chapter 1

Weight loss refers to the process of bringing about a reduction in total body mass, which is often accomplished by making adjustments to one's eating habits, level of physical activity, and many other aspects of one's lifestyle. Since being overweight may lead to a variety of health issues and chronic illnesses, it is essential for obtaining and keeping an overall healthy and well-balanced state of being. The advantages of losing weight include an improvement in both one's physical and mental health, as well as an increase in one's energy and vitality, a reduction in one's chance of developing chronic illnesses, and an overall rise in quality of life.

A persistent effort is required for successful weight reduction, which includes maintaining a nutritious diet, engaging in regular exercise, and making constant adjustments to one's lifestyle. Before beginning any program to lose weight, it is essential to discuss the plan with a qualified medical practitioner to verify that the plan is both safe and successful.

Losing weight is essential for several reasons, including the following:

1. Being overweight or obese may put one at risk for a variety of health conditions, including high blood pressure, stroke, heart disease, diabetes, and some forms of cancer. Losing weight can help improve one's physical health. Reducing weight is one of the best ways to enhance one's general physical health and cut one's chance of developing certain illnesses.

2. Reduced Risk of Anxiety, Depression, and Other Mood Disorders Excess weight is associated with an increased risk of developing anxiety, depression, and other mood disorders. A healthier body weight

may lead to increased self-esteem and confidence, as well as a more upbeat and optimistic attitude toward life.

3. Improved Energy and Vitality: Carrying extra weight may be physically demanding, which can contribute to weariness and lower energy levels. Losing weight can increase your energy levels and improve your vitality. Weight loss may result in increased levels of energy and vitality, making it simpler to participate in physically demanding activities and take pleasure in day-to-day living.

4. Obesity is a key risk factor for a variety of chronic illnesses, including heart disease, stroke, and diabetes. Losing weight may help reduce your chance of developing these conditions. The chance of developing certain illnesses and improving one's general health may both be improved by losing weight.

Weight loss may enhance the overall quality of life by lowering the amount of physical pain experienced, promoting mobility, and contributing to an overall sense of well-being.

The science of weight reduction is complex, but at its core, it revolves around striking a balance between the number of calories you take in and the number of calories you burn. If you take in more calories than you burn off each day, your body will store the surplus energy as fat, which will cause you to put on weight. When you do the opposite of what I just said and burn more calories than you take in, your body will start to burn fat for energy, which will result in weight reduction.

The pace and quantity of weight loss are both impacted by several different variables, including the following:

- BMR stands for "basal metabolic rate," which refers to the amount of energy that is expended by the body to carry out fundamental processes such as breathing, blood circulation, and temperature regulation. Individuals who have a greater basal metabolic rate burn more calories when they are at rest, making it simpler for them to reduce their overall body fat percentage.

- Exercise and other forms of physical activity assist to speed up the pace at which calories are burned, which in turn contributes to weight reduction. Weight reduction may be affected by several factors, including the kind of exercise performed, how strenuously, and how often.

Diet: Both what you eat and what you drink have an effect on your ability to lose weight. Losing weight may be accomplished by eating a nutritious diet that has an appropriate mix of nutrients and consuming fewer calories than you burn every day.

The fact that some individuals have a more difficult time losing weight than others owing to their genetic composition indicates that genetics play a part in the process of weight reduction.

Hormones: Hormones such as insulin, cortisol, and leptin may influence weight loss by controlling metabolism, hunger, and fat storage. Hormones such as these can have an impact on how much weight a person loses.

Losing weight has several advantages for one's health and young appearance, including the following:

1. Decreased Risk of Chronic Disorders Being overweight or obese is a risk factor for a variety of chronic illnesses, including heart disease, stroke, diabetes, and some forms of cancer. Nevertheless, maintaining a healthy weight may reduce your chance of developing these diseases. The chance of developing certain illnesses and improving one's general health may both be affected by weight loss.

2. Reduced Risk of Heart Disease and Stroke Lowering one's weight may have the effect of lowering one's blood pressure, which in turn decreases the chance of developing heart disease and stroke.

3. Improved Insulin Sensitivity and Management of Blood Sugar Reducing weight may enhance insulin sensitivity and improve control of blood sugar,

which can reduce the risk of diabetes and other metabolic illnesses.

4. Increased Joint Comfort and Stability Carrying extra weight puts additional pressure on the joints, which may cause discomfort and pain in the joints. The condition of your joints and the amount of discomfort you experience may improve if you lose weight.

5. Improved Energy and Vitality: Carrying extra weight may be physically demanding, which can contribute to weariness and lower energy levels. Losing weight can increase your energy levels and improve your vitality. Weight loss may result in increased levels of energy and vitality, making it simpler to participate in physically demanding activities and take pleasure in day-to-day living.

The quality of your sleep may improve as a result of your weight loss, as well as your reduced chance of developing sleep apnea and other sleep disorders.

Reduced Risk of Anxiety, Depression, and Other Mood Disorders Excess weight is associated with an increased risk of anxiety, depression, and other mood disorders. A healthier body weight may lead to increased self-esteem and confidence, as well as a more upbeat and optimistic attitude on life.

Anti-Aging Benefits: Research has shown that losing weight may reduce the process of aging by lowering oxidative stress and inflammation in the body. This results in a more youthful look as well as improvements in health.

Chapter 2

Achieving and maintaining a healthy weight requires first and foremost an awareness and comprehension of one's own body and weight. To have a better understanding of your body and its weight, consider the following:

Do a Body Mass Index (BMI) calculation. Your BMI score is a measurement of your body fat that is dependent on your height and weight. It is used as a tool for determining if a person has an abnormally low weight, an abnormally high weight, an overweight weight, or an obese weight. On the other hand, it is not an entirely accurate measurement since it does not take into consideration elements such as the amount of muscle mass or the overall composition of the body.

Determine your Body Composition The term "body composition" refers to the proportion of a person's body that is composed of fat vs muscle. Even if their body mass index falls within the normal range, a person who has a high proportion of body fat may nevertheless be considered overweight or obese. Bioelectrical impedance analysis (BIA), also known as skinfold thickness measures, and dual-energy x-ray absorptiometry are three of the many methods that may be used to determine an individual's body composition (DXA).

Keep an eye on your caloric balance. Your caloric balance is the difference between the number of calories you take in and the number of calories you burn. If you take in more calories than you burn, you will put on weight; on the other hand, if you burn more calories than you take in, you will reduce the amount of weight you carry. Maintaining a healthy weight might be easier if you keep track of the calories you consume and the calories you burn.

Increase the Rate at Which You Burn Calories Your metabolism is the pace at which your body uses up calories. If your metabolism is working more efficiently, you will be able to burn more calories and shed more pounds more quickly. It is possible to speed up your metabolism by engaging in regular physical activity, maintaining a healthy diet, and receiving enough rest.

Pay Attention to Hormones Hormones such as insulin, cortisol, and leptin may impact weight growth and weight reduction by controlling metabolism, hunger, and the storage of fat in the body. Pay Attention to Hormones You may reach and maintain a healthy weight by keeping track of your hormone levels and making adjustments to your lifestyle to bring them into harmony.

Consider Altering Your Lifestyle Several aspects of one's lifestyle, such as one's food, level of physical activity, level of stress, amount of sleep, and smoking habits, may all have an impact on weight growth or reduction. You may reach and maintain a healthy weight by making good adjustments to your lifestyle, which can help you lose weight.

One's health and well-being need to maintain a healthy weight throughout their lifetime. Nonetheless, obtaining and maintaining a healthy weight may be difficult, particularly in light of the abundance of contradictory information and trend diets that are now available. It is necessary to get an understanding of your body and weight to achieve long-term success in managing your weight.

If you have an awareness of the elements that influence your weight, such as your body composition, metabolism, hormones, and lifestyle, you will be able to make educated choices about your eating and exercise routines, which will allow you to attain and maintain a healthy weight.

In this process, it is vital to approach weight reduction healthily and sustainably rather than attempting to obtain immediate results by taking harsh measures. This is because healthy weight loss is more likely to result in long-term success. Getting tailored advice on how to achieve and maintain a healthy weight may also be obtained via consultation with a healthcare expert, such as a registered dietitian or a physician.

The body mass index, often known as BMI, and the percentage of total body fat are two typical metrics that are used to evaluate an individual's weight and body composition. A brief explanation of each follows:

The Body Mass Index (BMI) is a measurement of a person's body fat that takes into account both their height and weight. To determine it, divide a person's weight in kilograms by their height in meters squared. The result is the body mass index. A person's status as underweight, normal weight, overweight, or obese may be deduced by their body mass index (BMI). The body mass index (BMI) is a metric that may help monitor population trends; nevertheless, it is not without its flaws since it does not take into consideration aspects such as muscle mass or body composition.

The term "body fat percentage" refers to the amount of fat in the body in comparison to other types of tissue, such as bone and muscle. Even if their body mass index falls within the normal range, a person who has a high proportion of body fat may nevertheless be considered overweight or obese. Bioelectrical impedance analysis (BIA), also known as skinfold thickness measures, and dual-energy x-ray absorptiometry are three of the many methods that may be used to determine a person's proportion of body fat (DXA). If you want a more precise picture of your body composition, measuring your body fat % rather than just your BMI is the way to go.

Both genetics and lifestyle factors contribute to the accumulation of excess fat in the body. A brief explanation of each follows:

Genes: There is a possibility that some individuals have genes that make them more likely to put on weight than others. A person's metabolism, appetite, and capacity to store fat may all be influenced, for instance, by certain gene variants. Yet, a person's weight is not just determined by their genes; lifestyle variables such as their nutrition and the amount of physical exercise they get may also have an effect on their weight.

Many aspects of an individual's lifestyle, particularly but not limited to the following, have been linked to an increased risk of obesity:

A poor diet may contribute to weight gain since it is common for poor diets to be heavy in calories, sweets, and bad fats.
Sedentary living: A sedentary lifestyle burns fewer calories than an active one, therefore it may contribute to weight gain. An active lifestyle can help burn more calories.
Overeating and disruption of hormones that govern metabolism and fat accumulation may both be caused by prolonged exposure to the stress hormone, cortisol.
Insufficiency of sleep: Lack of sleep may cause hormones that govern hunger and metabolism to become imbalanced, which can contribute to weight gain.

A number of medical problems, such as hypothyroidism and polycystic ovarian syndrome (PCOS), have been linked to increased body fat and weight gain.

Chapter 3

A long time ago, there lived a lady by the name of Sarah who was dissatisfied with both her weight and her general state of health. In the past, she had attempted a variety of diets and short solutions, but nothing ever seemed to work for her in the long run. Sarah made the decision one day to adopt a new strategy and to concentrate on developing a healthy lifestyle in order to lose weight.

Her first step was to schedule an appointment with a qualified dietician, who assisted her in formulating a healthy meal plan by recommending that she consume an abundance of fruits, vegetables, lean proteins, and whole grains. In addition, Sarah has begun keeping a food journal in which she records her meals as well as any snacks that she consumes.

After that, Sarah made it a point to include time every day for vigorous exercise as part of her regimen. She started out by going for walks every day, and over time, she built up both the intensity of her exercises and the length of time she spent doing them. In addition to that, she began going to yoga classes twice a week in order to reduce the effects of stress and increase her flexibility.

Sarah focused her attention not just on her nutrition and her exercise routine, but also on other aspects of her lifestyle, such as obtaining adequate sleep and learning to manage her stress. She began meditating and using other mindfulness practices to assist her in better managing her stress and enhancing her general health and well-being.

Over the course of time, Sarah saw considerable changes in both her weight and her general health. She was able to keep her good habits up for a longer period of time, which contributed to her increased levels of energy, strength, and self-assurance. Sarah was successful in achieving her weight reduction objectives and improving her general quality of life by placing more of an emphasis on developing a healthy lifestyle rather than looking for a fast cure.

To successfully lose weight and maintain a healthy weight, it is necessary to include in one's lifestyle a variety of healthy behaviors, including good eating habits, regular physical exercise, and other lifestyle variables. The following is an explanation of each component:

1. Adopting Good Eating Habits
   Adopting healthy eating habits is vital for obtaining and maintaining a healthy weight. This involves eating a balanced diet that consists of a range of foods that are rich in nutrients. This

involves ingesting a large number of fresh fruits and vegetables, as well as whole grains, lean proteins, and healthy fats while reducing the amount of processed and high-calorie meals you consume.

2. Participation in Regular Physical Activity Taking part in regular physical exercise may assist in the burning of calories and the improvement of general health. This may include things like brisk walking, running, cycling, strength training, and yoga, among other activities. It is advised that one strives for at least 150 minutes of aerobic activity per week at a moderate level, in addition to two days per week of strength training.

3. A Healthy Weight May Also Be Achieved and Maintained Through Other Lifestyle Factors Other lifestyle

variables such as managing stress, getting an adequate amount of sleep, and cutting down on alcohol intake can all play a part in obtaining and maintaining a healthy weight. Consuming an excessive amount of alcohol may lead to weight gain in addition to long-term stress and a lack of sleep, all of which can wreak havoc on the hormones that control appetite and metabolism.

All of them are essential components of a healthy lifestyle that should be included to successfully lose weight. The following is a concise explanation of each:

Exercise and other forms of physical activity: Engaging in regular forms of physical exercise is necessary for both the maintenance of a healthy weight and one's general health. Calories may be burned, cardiovascular health can be improved, and muscle can be built by participating in physical activities such as walking, running, cycling, strength training, and yoga.

Nutrition and healthy eating habits: To achieve and maintain a healthy weight, it is essential to consume a diet that is both well-rounded and diverse in terms of the types of foods that are rich in nutrients. This involves ingesting a large number of fresh fruits and vegetables, as well as whole grains, lean proteins, and healthy fats while reducing the amount of processed and high-calorie meals you consume.

Sleep and rest: Obtaining adequate quality sleep is vital for regulating hormones that govern hunger and metabolism, as well as for one's general health and sense of well-being. Sleep deprivation may have negative effects on hormone levels. The average adult needs between 7 and 9 hours of sleep per night.

The management of stress Long-term stress may cause disruptions in hormones that govern hunger and metabolism, which can lead to an increase in body fat. The management of stress via practices such as meditation, yoga, or deep breathing may assist in preventing unhealthy habits like overeating and promoting general health and well-being.

Chapter 4

The process of reaching and maintaining a healthy weight via the implementation of lifestyle modifications that are long-term and sustainable is the goal of effective weight reduction. Weight loss may have many positive effects on one's health, including lowering the chance of developing chronic illnesses, increasing one's mobility and flexibility, and enhancing one's sense of self-worth. Losing weight, on the other hand, may be difficult and calls for an all-encompassing strategy that involves developing good eating habits, maintaining a regular exercise routine, and learning how to better handle stress.

It is essential to approSuccessful weight reduction is not only about hitting a specific number on the scale or fitting into a lower size of clothes. It is about enhancing your entire health and well-being via sustainable lifestyle modifications that you can maintain long-term. This demands a change in mentality from short-term diets or fads to a long-term strategy that focuses on creating healthy habits.each weight reduction with the mentality that one can successfully accomplish their goals.

A diet that is both nutritious and well-balanced is one of the most important factors in a successful weight reduction program. This involves consuming a wide range of foods that are rich in nutrients, such as fruits, vegetables, whole grains, lean proteins, and healthy fats while minimizing the consumption of processed meals and foods that are high in calories. It is also vital to control portion sizes and develop mindful eating practices to prevent overeating.

Effective weight reduction also requires regular physical exercise. Calories may be burned, cardiovascular health can be improved, and muscle can be built by participating in physical activities such as walking, running, cycling, strength training, and yoga. It is advised to strive for at least 150 minutes of moderate-intensity aerobic activity each week, coupled with activities to develop muscle. Each week of aerobic activity of moderate intensity, in addition to strength training activities to build muscle.

Obtaining adequate quality sleep and controlling stress are other crucial components of healthy weight reduction. Prolonged stress may cause disruptions in hormones that govern hunger and metabolism, which can result in increased body fat. The management of stress via practices such as meditation, yoga, or deep breathing may aid in preventing unhealthy habits like overeating as well as promoting general health and well-being. Moreover, obtaining adequate quality sleep is vital for regulating hormones that affect hunger and metabolism, as well as for general health and well-being.

Successful weight reduction involves a holistic strategy that addresses both physical and emotional wellness.
The following is a list of methods that have been shown to effectively aid in weight loss:

Have objectives that are both attainable and reasonable. Doing so may help you stay motivated and on track with your weight reduction efforts. A weight reduction of one to two pounds each week is recommended since it is healthy and may be maintained over time.

Establish a calorie deficit: For weight loss, you need to ensure that you expend more calories than you take in daily. This may be accomplished by committing to good eating patterns and engaging in regular physical exercise consistently.

Maintain a record of the food that you eat. Maintaining a food journal or utilizing an app that tracks calories will assist you in being responsible and attentive to the food choices that you make. It is also able to assist in the identification of locations in which modifications may be required.

Concentrate on foods high in nutrient density: Consuming a diet that is abundant in foods high in nutrient density, such as fruits, vegetables, whole grains, lean protein, and healthy fats, can help you feel full and satisfied for longer, in addition to providing essential nutrients for overall health.

Include some kind of physical activity in your daily routine. Maintaining a regular exercise program may assist in the burning of calories and the improvement of general health. Strive for at least 150 minutes of aerobic activity each week at a low level, and be sure to include strength training activities so that you may gain muscle.

Obtain enough sleep: Having adequate quality sleep is vital for regulating hormones that govern hunger and metabolism. This may be accomplished by getting sufficient amounts of sleep. The average adult needs between 7 and 9 hours of sleep per night.

Take steps to manage your stress: Prolonged stress may cause disruptions in hormones that govern appetite and metabolism, which can contribute to an increase in body fat. It is possible to reduce the risk of compulsive eating and improve one's general health and well-being by practicing stress-reduction methods such as yoga, meditation, or deep breathing.

Chapter 5

While attempting to reduce their body fat, many individuals find that they run across a number of obstacles along the way. These are the following:

A deficiency of motivation It may be challenging to maintain one's motivation, particularly when it seems that one is making very little progress. To get beyond this, you should strive to conquer it by making objectives that are within your reach, measuring your progress, and enjoying your victories along the way. You may also keep yourself motivated by enlisting the help of your family and friends or by becoming a member of a support group.

It is natural to feel cravings and hunger while making dietary changes since your body adjusts to the new nutrients it is receiving. To get around this, consider increasing the amount of foods in your diet that are high in protein and fiber, since these nutrients may make you feel more full and content. In addition, don't keep bad foods in the home and make sure you have healthy snacks and meals planned ahead of time so you don't give in to your desires.

Lack of time: It may be difficult for many individuals to find the time to work out or prepare nutritious meals. You may get around this challenge by including some kind of physical exercise into your daily routine. For example, you might choose to use the stairs rather than the elevator, or you could take a stroll during your lunch break. You may also try doing your food preparation on the weekends so that you have less work to do during the week.

It is very uncommon for people who are trying to lose weight to reach a point when they are unable to make further progress despite their continuing efforts. To get around this, consider switching up your workout regimen, modifying your diet to incorporate a wider variety of foods, or cutting down on the number of calories you eat every day.

Pressure from friends and family as well as from other people in your social circle might make it harder to maintain a healthy lifestyle. Social gatherings. To get around this challenge, discuss your objectives and limits with the people in your immediate environment, and look for physically active pursuits that can serve as an acceptable replacement for more conventional forms of social interaction, such as organizing a hike in place of a get-together for drinks.

While attempting to lose weight, one of the most difficult challenges is learning how to control one's appetites and emotional eating. The following are some ways that might assist in the management of these issues:

Get an understanding of the underlying cause: It is necessary to have an understanding of the underlying causes of cravings and emotional eating before you can successfully control these behaviors. Do you eat because you are bored, under stress, or because of some other emotional trigger? When you have gained an understanding of the underlying reason, you can then begin to formulate ways to deal with it.

Managing cravings and eating out of emotion may be effectively controlled by planning nutritious meals and snacks. This is one of the most successful strategies. This may help you avoid eating out on impulse and provide you with alternatives that are better to resort to when you have cravings.

It may be helpful to become more aware of your thoughts and feelings if you practice mindfulness, which can be accomplished via activities such as meditation or exercises that include deep breathing. This may help you realize when you are feeling cravings or emotional triggers and allow you to take actions to control them before they cause you to overeat.

Distract yourself: When you feel a pang of hunger coming on, it might be good to engage in other activities, such as going for a walk, phoning a friend, or participating in a hobby. This may assist in taking your attention off of food and lessen the desire that you have to consume it.

It may be good to seek the assistance of a professional, such as a registered dietitian or therapist if you discover that despite your best efforts, you continue to struggle with cravings and emotional eating. If this is the case, it may be helpful to seek the support of a professional.

It is vital to address any medical conditions that may be contributing to or hurting your ability to lose weight when it comes to weight loss since these issues may make it more difficult to lose weight. The following are some medical conditions that may impede weight reduction and the solutions to those conditions:

Thyroid issues: Thyroid conditions, such as hypothyroidism, may make it challenging to maintain a healthy weight. See your healthcare practitioner for testing and treatment if you have any concerns that you may be suffering from a thyroid problem.

Sleep apnea may make it harder to lose weight and can lead to weight gain. Sleep apnea can also cause weight gain. If you think you may have sleep apnea, you should discuss diagnostic and treatment options with your healthcare professional as soon as possible.

Medication: Some drugs, such as antidepressants and steroids, are known to promote weight gain in certain people. Have a conversation with your healthcare physician about any drugs you are currently taking and whether or not they might be affecting your capacity to shed excess pounds.

Polycystic ovarian syndrome (PCOS) is a condition in which there are hormonal abnormalities, which may make it difficult to lose weight. If you think you may have PCOS, you should discuss diagnosis and treatment options with your healthcare professional as soon as possible.
Diabetes: Diabetes that is not under control might make it very difficult to reduce weight. If you have diabetes, you must engage with your healthcare practitioner to monitor your blood sugar levels and design a weight reduction strategy that is both safe and successful.

Chapter 6

It might be just as difficult to keep the weight off as it was to lose it in the first place. It is crucial to design a strategy to maintain your weight reduction and avoid regaining the weight after you have met your weight loss objectives. This will help you keep the weight off. This might include implementing healthy behaviors into your lifestyle, such as going to the gym on a regular basis, adopting good eating habits, learning strategies to handle stress, and getting enough sleep. It may also include keeping a close eye on your progress and modifying your strategy in accordance with the requirements of the situation. You will not only be able to realize your objectives regarding weight reduction, but you will also be able to maintain a healthy weight and make improvements to both your general health and well-being.

Developing habits that can be maintained over time is essential to the effectiveness of weight reduction efforts in the long run. The following are some suggestions for developing a lifestyle that is more environmentally friendly:

Establishing goals that can be achieved is the first step in the process of setting realistic objectives. Try to avoid establishing objectives that are impossible to achieve since doing so might lead to frustration and disappointment.

Find activities you enjoy: Include in your daily routine the kinds of enjoyable physical activities that you do, such as going for a walk, riding a bike, or going swimming. A consistent workout regimen will be much simpler to maintain as a result of this.

Eat with an awareness of both what you are eating and why you are eating it. This is the practice of mindful eating. Put your focus on consuming entire, nutrient-dense meals that can both offer fuel for your body and help you feel full.

Create healthy routines: Create healthy routines that you can sustain over a long period, such as meal planning, having nutritious snacks on hand, and drinking a lot of water.

Take steps to manage your stress. Stress may play a role in weight gain and can make it more challenging to lead a healthy lifestyle. Make stress management practices a regular part of your routine. Some examples of stress management practices are meditation, yoga, and deep breathing exercises.

Obtaining appropriate rest Getting the recommended amount of sleep each night is critical for maintaining a healthy weight. Try to get between seven and eight hours of sleep per night.

You may establish a lifestyle that is sustainable and promotes long-term success in weight reduction if you include these guidelines into your daily routine and make them a part of your habit.

Recognizing and honoring your accomplishments along the way is an essential component of leading a healthy lifestyle and keeping the motivation necessary to keep working toward your weight reduction objectives. You should celebrate your victory in one of the following ways:

Establish milestones: Along the road, establish certain benchmarks for success, and celebrate each one as it is achieved. For instance, make a big deal out of the fact that you've dropped five or ten pounds or that you've been working out regularly for a certain amount of time.

Reward yourself: When you accomplish a significant goal, reward yourself by doing something nice for yourself, such as getting a massage, purchasing new exercise gear, or eating a nutritious meal at your favorite restaurant.

Show your loved ones and friends how far you've come by discussing your accomplishments with them and letting them know how far you've come. Celebrate with a meal or activity that is good for you and that you all like doing together.

Take some time to think about how far you've gone and how much effort you've put into achieving your objectives, and give yourself credit for the effort you've already put out.

Instead of using food as a reward, consider rewarding yourself with non-food things such as a new book, movie, or anything else that you take pleasure in.

You may maintain your motivation and keep making headway toward your weight reduction objectives by recognizing the victories you've already achieved along the way. It is important to remember to appreciate even the smallest of victories and to take pleasure in the process of being healthier and happy.

Obstacles are an inevitable part of the process of losing weight, but they have the potential to be very unpleasant and demotivating. The following is a list of suggestions for overcoming obstacles:

Be sympathetic and nice to yourself. It is essential to be compassionate and kind toward oneself while you are going through a difficult time. Try to stop yourself from having negative thoughts and keep in mind that failures are a natural part of the process.

You need to change your thinking so that you don't perceive setbacks as failures but rather as chances to learn and develop from the experience. Examine your strategy in search of ways to improve it and get closer to achieving your objectives.

Determine the reason: One should make an effort to determine the root cause of the problem, which might be a lack of motivation, stress, or a particular trigger. After you've determined what caused the problem, you'll be able to take action to fix it and avoid similar obstacles in the future.

Go back on the right path and do not allow temporary obstacles to derail your success. Get your life back on track as quickly as you can by rededicating yourself to your healthy routines and making progress toward your objectives.

Do not be hesitant to seek help from friends, family, or even a healthcare professional. Get support, and do not be afraid to do so. Having a network of people who have your back might help keep you motivated and accountable.

You will be able to overcome obstacles and keep moving forward in the direction of achieving your weight reduction goals if you handle setbacks with compassion and take preventative measures. Don't forget to exercise some patience.

It may be difficult to make progress with your health objectives, but you must maintain your dedication to the process of becoming a better and happier version of yourself. Remind yourself to work towards your objectives in the baby stages and to enjoy even the little victories along the road. You shouldn't allow failures to impede your development; rather, you should utilize them as chances to learn and grow from your experiences. When you find yourself in a difficult situation, look for assistance, and surround yourself with encouraging people who can keep you motivated and on course. You will be able to attain your weight reduction objectives and live your best life if you put an emphasis on your health and make long-term, sustainable adjustments to your lifestyle. Never stop moving , ahead and always have faith in yourself

This table of contents covers a range of topics related to weight loss, including the science of weight loss, understanding your body and weight, building a healthy lifestyle, effective weight loss strategies, overcoming common challenges, maintaining weight loss, and celebrating success. In conclusion, this table of contents covers a range of topics related to weight loss, including the science of weight loss, understanding your body and weight, building a healthy lifestyle, and building a healthy lifestyle. Each chapter provides insightful information and useful advice from industry professionals to assist you in achieving your weight reduction goals and maintaining a healthy lifestyle. Keep in mind that getting rid of excess weight is a process that requires time, patience, and dedication to see results. You may create changes in your life that are lasting and bring about a better and healthier version of yourself if you have the correct mentality, enough support, and good habits.